GW00659197

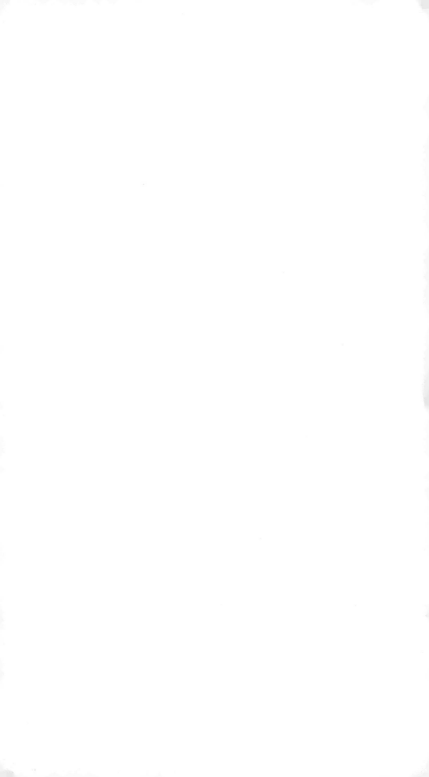

RMJ DONALD

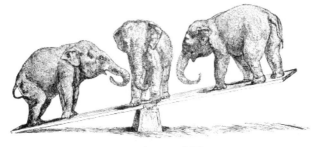

Fine Books and Plays

P.O. Box 8
Barrington, NH
03825

RMJ DONALD
Fine Books and Plays
P.O. Box 8 • Barrington • NH 03825

ESSENTIAL LESSAC
Copyright © 2014 Deborah Kinghorn

ISBN 978-0-9884982-1-1

Book Design
RMJ DONALD, LLC

Available Worldwide

Dedicated to my husband, Jeffrey, without whose encouragement, advice, skill, and love, this book would never have been realized.

We wish to acknowledge the following people for their direct and indirect contributions to this book: Michael Lessac, Sue Ann Park, Nancy Krebs, Barry Kur, Dick Cuyler, Edward Edwards, Crystal Robbins, Maria Evegard, and the Certified Trainers and Practitioners of the Lessac Training and Research Institute.

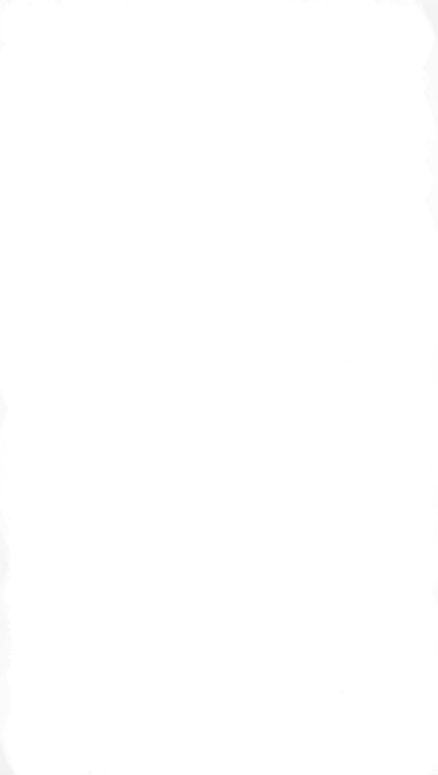

ESSENTIAL LESSAC
Honoring the familiar in

body
mind
spirit

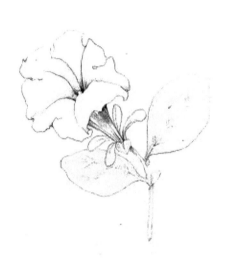

Content

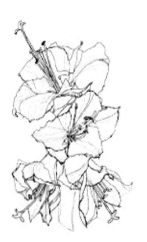

Forward

An Invitation from Arthur Lessac

When I was two and half years old, my parents divorced and thereafter, for reasons unknown to me, I had little or no contact with either of them. This, of course, had a profound effect on me. First, I had no real home. I moved between relatives or friends of relatives, always having shelter, but never having a family or a home. For much of my early life, I was alone. I have no regrets about this now. I believe it is what led me to the discoveries which later shaped my research, work, and, eventually, brought me to love and happiness.

In order to survive, I had to find a way of feeling good. Since I could not rely on the outer environment, it had to come from my own inner environment. Singing was my first discovery; I realized that whenever I sang, I felt good. And I found myself almost always humming or singing.

It became my natural path to connecting with other people.

Although I constantly hummed to myself, it wasn't enough. Wherever I went, even when carrying my satchel on my shoulder to each of my new addresses, my body, a small one, seemed to turn itself into a leprechaun, light-footed, nimble, full of dance.

So I hummed or sang and at some point I realized that it not only felt good, but that it was a bridge to unexpected awareness and fresh inner feeling. It chased away fatigue, worry, concern, and it shook away all sense of negativity.

I did not sing because I knew it would make me feel better—I sang because my body wanted the comfort, joy, and, yes, even courage that were generated whenever my voice vibrated within me. I came to realize that it not only felt good, but that it was healthy. To this day, I ask myself and my students:

When you walk, do you feel like you're dancing?

When you talk, do you feel like you are singing?

As I grew into adulthood and began my formal study of voice and body work, this awareness carried into my clinical therapy studies, where I learned that tonal vibrations could have remarkable healing qualities. My curiosity led me to ask: If making tone or singing can heal, what else can the body do for itself?

I began to study children and animals, and observed their movement to be without patterning or tension, and I began to understand how the body functions when it is free of stress and disease.

I marveled at the movement of Charlie, our cat, and at the beautiful clear tones made by my children, and the way in which they moved, stood, sat, and played. I understood from these observations that thinking was not involved—it was a feeling process. Children and animals simply respond to the inspiration of the moment. Eventually, I defined the feeling process as:

The means by which the energy called feeling is perceived in the inner environment and is used for wellness and awareness.

From that one realization grew a lifetime of exploration; a lifetime, too, of saying no to the poisons of the outer environment and yes to inner environment health.

Since my 20's (hence, for the last 80 years), I have used myself as a research subject upon whom to test my theories about the body's natural wisdom. As I integrated my findings into my teaching, I discovered that my conclusions were validated again and again by my students. They, too, found that the feeling process was a simple and direct way to teach themselves how to tap into the vast potential for wellness inside their bodies.

In 1984, I met the co-author of this book, Deborah Kinghorn. We immediately recognized in each other kindred spirits. In the last decade, we have spent hundreds of hours defining and challenging our understanding of the feeling process in ourselves, as well as exploring the natural effect of this process on our families, friends, and communities. This book represents our shared explorations and conclusions.

Since I am currently 101 years young, and she is half my age, I am happy to know that Deby will continue the research we have conducted together. In the writing of this book, we have chosen deliberately to use the word we. Some of the experiences are mine, some are Deby's; to whom they belong has no bearing on the experience itself.

That brings me to the purpose of our book, and how we suggest you use it.

You will learn to appreciate your innate body wisdom and its teachings. By listening to your body, you will learn to trust your inner voice rather than the dictates of the external world.

Through these personal discoveries, you will learn about and experience the power of sensation, vibration, and energy, which will promote a feeling of wellness and wholeness in you.

You will learn to differentiate the feeling process from patterns of thinking, which often cycle in endless loops and carry you nowhere. You will discover ways to rid yourself of the obstacles to joy, health, and wellness.

In Part One you will read about **Familiar Events,** which come from your behavior, and will be engaged to identify and expand your feeling process. For this reason, you will find the book full of short experiments and explorations. You don't have to be a scientist, doctor, or any other kind of practitioner to apply these simple concepts. Your body will lead you to the learning, and the chapters on creating a better world will invite you to expand your sense of well-being to others.

Finally, this book asks you to stop wishing or hoping for change from the outside. Inside of you is an environment full of intelligence and sensitivity—intrinsic body wisdom. This is an often unexplored wilderness for many of us. We invite you to wander in this wilderness with us and discover the health and wellness that is your natural state.

Arthur Lessac
August 2010

Part One: **PRECISE SENSATION**

The Feeling Process

Awareness that health is dependent on habits we control makes us the first generation in history that to a large extent determines its own destiny.

Jimmy Carter

Healthfulness—the state of being *full* of *health*—is an inner sensation. When you are full of health, you feel good.

When you pursue inner healthfulness, interesting things start to happen. External noise fades away and you can hear the soft voice of the body's native intelligence guiding you through your senses to a state of wellness.

When you feel good inside, you naturally want to do things that will keep you fit. You take joy in exercise and foods that provide nourishment. When you feel good, you enjoy life. You stay out of the doctor's office and off the psychiatrist's couch. By becoming aware of our physical inner sensations, we can learn about our needs and develop reliable means by which we experience the inner health that is essential to our being.

LEARNING THROUGH OUR SENSES

You have learned through your senses since you were a baby. Take crawling, for example. A baby begins by experimenting with her body—learning how to roll over, learning to push up with her arms and legs, and learning that putting one hand in front of the other causes the legs to follow, and suddenly, she is moving forward! Each step opens the way to the next step, and all are accomplished by following one sensation with the next one, and learning from the process. The baby may be struggling to crawl but, likely, is not *thinking* about each incremental effort in the endeavor, as one does as an adult. That is, the baby does not read the directions for crawling and think:

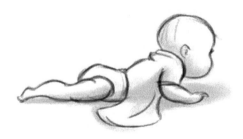

Okay, if I put this hand here, and follow up with this knee, I should be crawling!

More likely, there is simply joy in sensing and exploring. Everything in the baby's environment is registered and recorded—the texture of the carpet, the sensation of pulling and pushing, the sound of a dog barking nearby. Learning occurs continuously via sensation, exploration, and experimentation. As sensory learning accumulates, the baby feels subtler sensations, such as the calm that results from hearing a soothing tone of voice, which, in turn, stimulates feelings of love and safety. Inner sensing is the first part of the feeling process.

As elementary as this may seem, we are making it our business to separate even the simplest of sensations into separate parts in order to more richly rediscover what we assume we already know.

How often as adults have we sensed fear, loneliness, or even danger, yet go on to adopt behaviors that allow us to remain oblivious to such feelings?

If we allow ourselves to learn from our bodies, we can discover natural remedies for negativity and pain, and there would be no need to make ourselves oblivious to them.

Humming

Singing

Dancing

Rogers and Hammerstein have given us a memorable example of those very behaviors in these lyrics from *The King and I:*

> *Whenever I feel afraid*
>
> *I hold my head erect*
>
> *And whistle a happy tune*
>
> *So no one will suspect*
>
> *I'm afraid.*

Perhaps these lyrics are memorable because the sensations are familiar.

When you lengthen the spine *(hold my head erect)* and feel the movement of the facial muscles when *(whistling)* it is virtually impossible for your face or body to be frozen in fear. But, wait, there is more:

> *I whistle a happy tune*
>
> *And every single time*
>
> *The happiness in the tune*
>
> *Convinces me that I'm not afraid.*

Rogers and Hammerstein suggest you can change fear into ease without resorting to anything but a whistle—simple!

Because it is simple, we tend to be unconscious of the inclination and end up being oblivious to it.

The dividend to slowing down and examining these incremental actions is that we rediscover the healing qualities inherent in them.

Reclaim this natural way of learning and there is much that you can teach yourself that will lead to improved health. Another simple example:

When you wake up, do you yawn?

Do you also feel an impulse to stretch?

Could you go so far as to say that the body wants to yawn as much as the face does?

Muscle Yawn—let's coin that term.

Muscle Yawning with the whole body engages you in reaching, and that kind of movement invigorates. When you ***Muscle Yawn*** your body, you summon power not force.

We will discuss the difference between power and force in greater detail momentarily. It is enough, now, to stay with the yawning sensation which relaxes muscles and joints.

How does this relate to health? Let's break our discussion down into simple parts again and take a closer look.

❖ Yawning relaxes muscles and joints.

❖ Movement is easier.

❖ Posture improves.

❖ Breathing is deeper and more natural.

❖ Organ function improves.

❖ Energy and vitality increase.

What you learn from the feeling process can lead to better health, to a better sense of well-being, to a better life, perhaps even to a better world.

You don't need to buy a lot of equipment to start; you don't need to go to a special place of learning. You have only to go inside yourself, where you experience this so naturally every day that it is easy to overlook and even discount it.

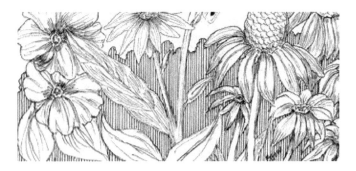

A Whole New World

A man is not rightly conditioned until he is a happy, healthy, and prosperous being; and happiness, health, and prosperity are the result of a harmonious adjustment of the inner with the outer of the man with his surroundings.

James Allen

The Environments

You are living and functioning in two different worlds. One is very familiar to you; the other is likely a place outside your everyday awareness.

Let's call these two worlds the inner and the outer environments. On the one hand, there is the huge outer environment, with everything and everyone else in it, its widely varied cultures, its unexplored territories, its powerful energy forces (nuclear, electrical, solar, water, etc.), and its conditioning and patterning, which shape the way you think and act.

On the other hand, there is your vast inner environment, with only you in it, your personality, your unexplored inner wilderness, and your intrinsic body energies which promote vitality and create health and well-being.

Poisons

While there are healthful elements in the outer environment, such as eating good foods, breathing oxygen, and laughing with friends and loved ones, there are unhealthy elements, too, such as the chemical additives in processed foods, the pollution of air and water, and fear, suspicion, even hatred of those who are different from us. The problem is that these unhealthy elements do not stay in the outer environment. They find their way into your inner environment, where they can do a great deal of damage. They act like poisons.

Antidote

The antidote to such poison lies within your inner environment—a body of systems that are likely not completely familiar to you, though you have probably heard some of the names:

- ○ Cellular
- ○ Circulatory
- ○ Digestive
- ○ Endocrine

- o Integumentary
- o Nervous
- o Musculoskeletal
- o Respiratory
- o Sensory
- o Urinary

You don't think about their functioning, but the processes of these systems are taking place every second of your life. They give you information without conscious awareness.

There are even subtler processes of the inner environment, some of which are:

- Consciousness
- Creativity
- Emotion
- Imagination
- Rhythm

These also provide information on the conscious, sub-conscious, and unconscious levels.

Poisons such as air and noise pollution, chemical/industrial waste, etc., make the outer environment uninhabitable.

Likewise, anger, hate, greed, jealousy, fear, etc., are poisons that make the inner environment uninhabitable.

While we rely on ecological watch-dog individuals and groups to alert us to poisons in the outer environment, the only ecological watch-dog for our inner environment is ourselves.

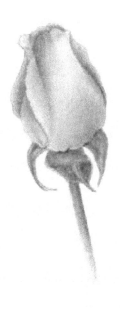

The Familiar Event

Tell me and I'll forget; show me and I may remember; involve me and I'll understand.

Chinese Proverb

Rediscovering the body's natural resources begins with a simple step: finding a **Familiar Event**.

Familiar Events are actions performed with ease thanks to talent or skill, and are, thus, likely pleasurable, graceful, and efficient. They are a healthy use of the body.

Smelling a lovely fragrance is an instinctive action, whether it is a flower, a cup of coffee, or your favorite perfume. Let's use it to better understand the concept of Familiar Event and how it can help us learn.

Pleasurable Smelling

- You are attracted by the fragrance of a lovely flower. Bend over, cup the flower in both hands, and inhale the fragrance as if you are doing it for the first time.

- Do it again, but this time, enjoy the fragrance. Do not rush the experience.

- Again, and this time, love the enjoyment of the fragrance.

- Finally, repeat the last step and become aware of your body's response to it.

Each time you smell the flower you feel more expansion in the torso, from the sides to the lower back and maybe even all the way up the back, creating a natural expansion of the thoracic cavity *(chest)*.

What you don't feel are your shoulders lifting up *(an unnatural action for breathing)*, nor expansion only in the front of your body, in the belly area, or lifting of your chest *(a very shallow way of breathing.)*

You can fill yourself from bottom to top with that fragrance, yet there is no strain or force, just the enjoyment of smelling something pleasurable.

This is the sensation of the body's natural way of breathing. If you feel that expansion in response to smelling something fragrant, whether you take a large breath or a small one, you will always get a healthy breath.

Take note that the Familiar Event of pleasurable smelling has given you information about natural breathing.

Again, let's not stumble over or dismiss the importance of the Familiar Event with the assumption that it is so simple as to go without saying. Most of us do not breathe well.

Not breathing well acts as yet another poison to the inner environment. It can lead to high blood pressure, hypertension, anxiety, depression, insomnia, chronic pain, and to premature aging.

You have probably guessed already that we have the remedy easily within our grasp by returning to the Familiar Event of pleasurable smelling.

Organic Instruction

Using the Familiar Event led to the discovery that if we smell the flower instead of trying to control our breath, we can achieve the most natural way of breathing without effort. Thus, Familiar Event leads to Organic Instruction.

Organic Instruction is exactly what it sounds like—the body teaching you instead of you attempting to exert control over your body.

Organic can also mean healthy, much like the difference between organic and processed foods.

Organic Instruction, then, is healthy self-teaching. It creates balance, rhythm, and inspires well-being in the body. Non-organic instructions can create conflict and confusion in your body.

For example, you want to be louder. A non-organic instruction would be: *Throw your voice to the back wall.*

The voice cannot be thrown like a ball. To try to do so results in force, hoarseness, fatigue and strain.

An Organic Instruction instead might be*: Feel the vibrations of your voice inside your head.*

This is a direction which does not confuse the body, so there is no force or strain, merely the pleasure of feeling the sensation of your voice. You will be heard without self-inflicted damage.

Organic Instruction produces experience from the Familiar Event. Having learned what optimum breath feels like from smelling the flower, you can train yourself to recreate that feeling whenever you breathe, whether through your nose or through your mouth.

- Feel the sensations of breathing as you felt them when smelling the flower, but now, stand up straight.

Did you feel as much expansion in your lower torso? If not, why not? Let's look at posture.

- Once again, bend over to smell the flower.

Do you notice how much more expansion you feel in your lower torso?

What is different?

Note how far you bend, as much as a c-curve or as little as a gentle parenthesis in the spine.

- Now explore how you might carry this feeling of curvedness into your upright posture.

What do you find?

You discover that when your back is arched and tight, or when your chest is collapsed and you are slouching that you cannot get the full *smelling-the-flower-breath*.

You discover that the longer and looser you feel your spine to be, the more open and responsive your body is to the expansion that comes from smelling the flower.

If you breathe well, you stand well.

&

If you stand well, you breathe well.

From the Familiar Event of smelling the flower, you developed an Organic Instruction for good breathing. The sensations of good breathing form the Familiar Event from which you developed the Organic Instruction for good posture.

Each Organic Instruction becomes a Familiar Event for something else.

You are learning from sensation, you are self-teaching.

Your body knows what it needs

—listen to it—

It will help you become healthier

By finding a Familiar Event, and following the feeling process to Organic Instruction, you open the door to greater awareness of your body's natural functioning.

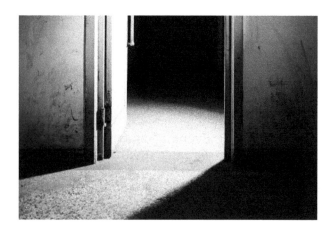

The Body's Pain Relievers

What we call pleasure, and rightly so, is the absence of all pain.

Cicero

If you had to *think* about what to do every time your body felt a pain or discomfort you would fall apart for lack of care! Thank goodness, the body knows how to take care of itself instinctively when something upsets it.

Imagine this scenario: you are walking along when suddenly you are pulled up short by a muscle cramp. What do you do?

Freeze?
•
Stretch?
•
Shake?

You have just experienced the body's natural pain relievers. It took more time to write them down than it does to actually feel them. But let's take them one by one.

o Freeze: You aren't really encased in ice; the feeling is more like suspending yourself, trying not to put weight on the cramp or engage in any sudden movement. Let's call this:

float

o Stretch: Lengthening or widening something without causing breakage or strain. When does the body do that naturally? Whenever you yawn; you extend or reach. We call this:

muscle yawn

o Shake: An intentional vigorous action that replicates vibration, already well-named. We'll call it:

shake

As if on automatic pilot, your body uses these actions to help relieve pain. You can engage them to help counteract stress, heaviness, floppiness, discomfort, pressure, tiredness or even lack of creative awareness.

These words all indicate a deadening of sensation, much like the effects of the anesthetic that you receive when you have an operation. From the Greek *anaisthetos*, its purpose is to make you feel nothing.

Opposite sensations would include:

Lightness
•
Weightlessness
•
Balance
•
Nimbleness
•
Creativity

Another legacy from the Greek language, a*esthetic* or its alternate *esthetic*, while referring to a sense of beauty, also means that which promotes sensation.

With that original meaning in mind, the three pain relievers—*float, muscle yawn,* and *shake* lead to what we will call: **Body Esthetics**.

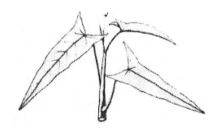

Experiment

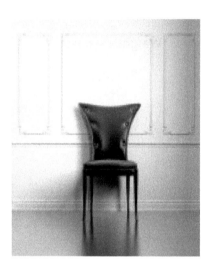

Sit in a chair.

- Imagine that you are sitting in a car and have been driving for quite a few hours. You are tired, and you stop to rest.

- Get up from your chair as if you are getting out of the car. Feel how stiff your muscles are.

- Muscle yawn throughout your body to relieve the stiffness. *(This is like the full body movement a cat indulges in when it wakes from sleep.)*

Notice how you want to reach further and further, and how good it feels. Also notice how the body feels fresher and energized.

- Muscle yawn one more time with your arms over your head. As you finish, turn off the yawn and let the body slowly return to its regular posture, allowing the arms to float down to your sides.

Notice how light yet how alert your body feels.

- *Shake* all through your body.

Notice the feeling of buzzing or vibrating inside the body when you stop the shake.

Do you see how easy it is to feel these pain relievers? Each one—muscle yawn, float, and shake—has distinctive qualities of movement and feeling associated with it. They help you feel good.

In addition to providing you with relief from tension and pain, the body's pain relievers also infuse you with energy.

Energy and relaxation are complementary opposites which function simultaneously to produce balance and ease. Think of them as yin and yang.

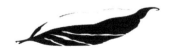

Their harmonious interaction produces a third energy, an offspring called: **Relaxer-Energizer.**

Energy and Relaxation

Relaxer-energizers are healthful, sensory experiences. They are not talents, skills, or techniques, and can't be pursued as such. For example, sighing pleasurably is a relaxer-energizer. The body does this when you need both the relaxation of the muscles and the energy from the oxygen that sighing provides.

Yet, when you force yourself to sigh, it is no longer effortless or pleasurable. You may have been told to take a deep breath upon feeling anxious or afraid or in pain. But that would not necessarily relax or energize you.

Why?

Because there is already significant tension in the very muscles you need to breathe, and forcing breath would only increase the tension.

However, if you ask yourself to smell the flower, the familiar, sensory experience of smelling something fragrant will immediately engage instinctive, optimal breathing, quickly calming you.

Let's take a moment to appreciate the difference between force and power as they are used in this book.

Force: *effort* **— *Power:*** *vigor*

***Force*:** *excessive* **— *Power*:** *efficient*

Power: *gathers* **— *Force:*** *consumes*

Power: *strengthens* **— *Force:*** *weakens*

Force is an anesthetic that produces tension and pain in the body. Power releases tension and stimulates sensation, making it a body esthetic.

Back to Relaxer-Energizers.

Recall that the body pain relievers relax us, as in the example of the muscle-cramp. We have explored how those same pain relievers served us upon getting out of the car. The key is that in relaxing, they release energy which invigorates.

Recasting and adding to them as actions now, our new list includes:

Yawning

Floating

Shaking

Humming

Sighing

Smiling

Singing

Laughing

Dancing

When these physical activities are organic, they are initiated on impulse stimulated by need and inspiration, rather than by intellectual choice.

The combination of breathing and posture is also a relaxer-energizer, as in the smelling the flower exploration. The inspiration and the long spine gave you both relaxation and energy at the same time. Smelling, of course, cannot occur without respiration (breathing).

The body's native rhythm, unencumbered by environmental distortion, is a sophisticated yet natural component of all movement and is a relaxer-energizer which affords an experience of body symmetry, balance, and expression.

Dancing as a Relaxer-Energizer

The most relaxing and invigorating kind of dancing is neither choreographed nor learned, it comes spontaneously from an impulse inside us.

- Play your favorite kind of music. Don't worry if it has a dance beat—just play whatever music you enjoy.

- Stand in the middle of the room. Close your eyes, and simply listen to the music.

- As you listen, feel the mood and rhythm of the music. Enjoy it.

- Allow your body to begin to move in any direction. It can be slight and it can start anywhere, with swaying from side to side or front to back, with an arm floating up, or with a toe tapping, etc.

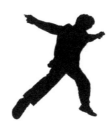

Once you feel the movement in your body, however light or gentle it may be, answer that movement with another part of your body. For example, if you are nodding your head, you might answer the head with a movement in your shoulders. You may find they even want to talk at the same time. Let them!

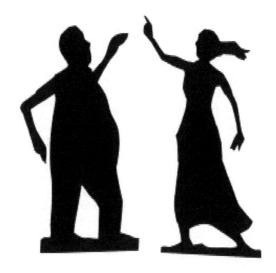

- Play with moving different parts of your body in the mood of the music, as if your body is holding a movement conversation with itself.

- Explore connecting some of these movements together, as if you are now creating longer sentences. You might even feel that you need to move your feet in order to experience more freedom.

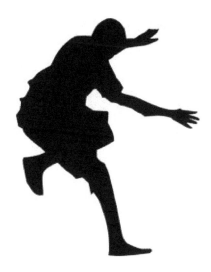

- Keep focused on enjoying the music you have chosen. Let your movement simply express that enjoyment.

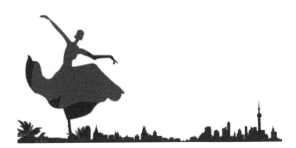

- When your music has finished, continue to feel it inside of you. Walk to the next room, feeling inside of you the personal rhythm you have just created. Let it affect the way you walk.

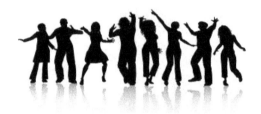

How do you feel? Invigorated, yet refreshed? Is there a smile on your face, or even inside of you? This is how a relaxer-energizer works. We are all capable of beautiful, personal dancing which is the origin of all folk dancing; in fact, of *all* dancing.

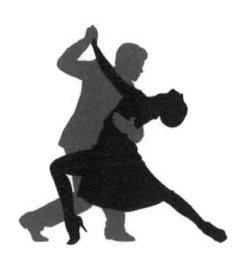

Laughing as a Relaxer-Energizer

We've all heard the phrase *Laughter is the best medicine*. It is well-known that laughter is healthy and can help prevent or treat a host of diseases and illnesses. It is reasonable to assume that everybody has experienced laughter. But can you laugh on demand? How do you laugh to heal yourself when you don't feel like laughing? First, you have to feel the sensation of laughter.

- Think of something you enjoy. It can be a person, an animal, a day at the beach, anything that gives you pleasure.

- Smile. Let the smile grow as you enjoy the thing that is giving you pleasure. Can you feel your smile not just in the lips, but in the eyes as well? Can you feel your face relaxing, opening, expanding?

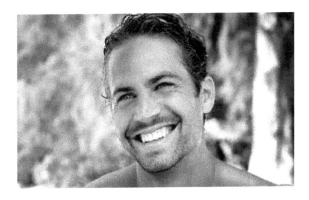

- Take a deep breath in. Hold it.

- Now, while still smiling, open your mouth and breathe out, but add some sound to it. Of course, *ha* is good, but it can be *hee* or *ho* or any vowel you want, or even an *n* or *ng* consonant. At the same time, start shaking the body. Shoulders are a good way to start, but it can come from any body shaking.

- Let the shaking break up the tone into little bursts, *he-he-he* or *hn-hn-hn,* and you will feel yourself beginning to laugh.

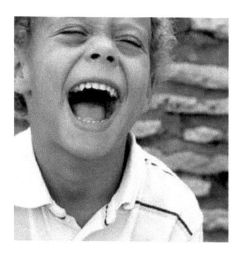

How much you laugh, or how far this experiment takes you, depends on how much you enjoy the thing you chose to think about. But even so, laughter has a life of its own. Once it starts, it can quickly grow, especially if it is shared with someone.

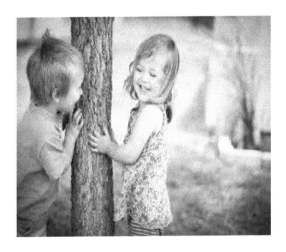

Laughing might not be the first thing you think of when you are stressed. But laughter is a combination of relaxed shaking and pleasurable sighing, two relaxer-energizers. Its action releases the body from tension, whether you know the tension is there or not. And while that release is happening, you are getting energized by the good feelings that come with the laughter. All of this is healthy for the body.

You have now felt the familiar events of the body's natural pain relievers and have experienced the relaxer-energizers.

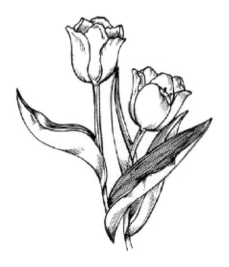

The Body NRGs

When you walk do you feel like you're dancing?

Arthur Lessac

Energy

All physical substance consists of matter, and all matter is in motion.

Energy is the capacity to cause change or to do work. It is engaged any time an alteration in matter occurs. Energy cannot be created or destroyed; it can only be transformed from one form into another.

Kinetic Energy
characterized by motion

Potential Energy
stored or dormant

As energy converts from potential to kinetic and back again, you can sense the ebb and flow of temperature changes and motion in your body. Playing baseball, riding a bike, or just walking are sensed as movement and any attendant changes in the temperature in your body are sensed, as well. Your breathing and the pumping of your heart can be felt, too, though on a subtler level of awareness.

Even more subtle is emotion. Love and hate produce physical and chemical changes in your body, both of which indicate kinetic energy.

Recall the pain relievers, yawning, shaking, and floating; all are movements which create different temperatures and sensations in your body. Whenever you engage them, you initiate change in your body's matter because you are using energy.

These three pain relievers now form the basis for our body's energy. We acknowledge that most physicists would look askance at our use of this terminology; therefore, we'll make our use distinct from the sciences by shortening it to **NRG.**

Our labels reflect the quality or the primary characteristic of the body's kinetic energy.

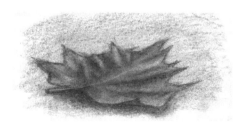

Rejuvenation

A young man studying at drama school in New York City in the early 1970's receives a free ticket to a Broadway concert given by the Atlantic City Steel Pier Band. He observes his fellow theatre-goers, most of them much older, being helped down the aisles, using canes and walkers, unable to walk unassisted.

As the band begins to play music of the 30's and 40's, he sees heads nodding in time, then shoulders beginning to keep the beat as well. Pretty soon, feet start tapping, and bodies begin to sway.

Almost magically by intermission, those who could not walk unassisted into the theatre discard their walkers and canes and are up and dancing together in the aisles. It is as if they had rediscovered the fountain of youth.

What could have caused this extraordinary rejuvenation? Was it, as many poets and philosophers have noted, the power of music?

Or was there something else?

How did those bodies, creaky and stiff with the aches and pains of age, suddenly find the springing step of youth?

The answer, it turns out, can be found in the body's NRG resources.

In your inner environment, you can experience and identify six different NRGs grouped as:

Body NRGs
Buoyancy
Radiancy
Potency

Vocal NRGs
Consonant
Structure
Tone

The pain relievers and the relaxer-energizers now become your familiar events to recognize these NRGs.

Buoyancy

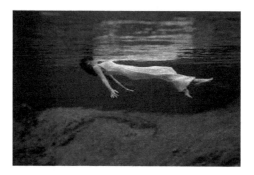

- You've finished the last assignment for your job and you can finally leave on vacation. You feel free as a bird, as light as a feather!

- You're floating in a pool, drifting without care, enjoying the sense of weightlessness

- You're tired but happy, slowly sinking into your pillow and gently drifting off to sleep.

All of the above situations are occurrences of buoyancy in everyday life.

Buoyancy is the organic instruction that evolves from the familiar event of floating.

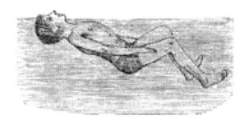

The feeling is analogous to floating in a pool or bathtub, where by filling your lungs with air you become lighter than the water you displace. Because water is denser than air, you can surrender your weight to it without fear of falling. Of course, you don't live in the water. But a simple isometric exercise will demonstrate that buoyancy can be felt when out of water as well.

Weightlessness

- Stand in an open doorway, or next to a smooth wall.

- Press the back of one wrist against the door frame or wall.

- Muscle yawn through that arm, enjoying the feeling of the yawn.

- Step lightly and quickly away from the door frame or wall and allow your arm to float up.

- Do the same with the other arm.

- Explore both sides at the same time. Enjoy the sensation.

The arm feels weightless, with the sense that there is no conscious use of your muscles. You know they are working, but you are not feeling the work. Buoyancy is dynamic relaxation. Feeling buoyancy creates the perception that movement can be virtually weightless and non-fatiguing.

From water to air

- Imagine that the air is like water—it has density and mass.

- Allow your arm to float up.

- With your arm, cut a swath through the air, parting the air molecules and feeling them close around your arm as you pass through them.

- Float the arm down.

Whether floating up like a helium-filled balloon, or gliding like a bird riding the currents of the air, or floating down like a weightless feather, the buoyancy sensation is often associated with feelings of relaxation, centeredness, hope, calm, peace, serenity, total awareness and connection with the inner world.

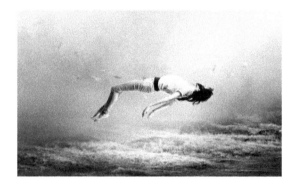

Did you know that astronauts gain up to two inches of height in space? Why? No gravity. They are weightless.

Here on earth, gravity exerts its force on you, compressing your spine. Buoyancy is a powerful anti-gravity NRG which can counteract that compression.

Buoyancy felt in your walk is a powerful protector of your joints. If you feel buoyancy, you can do anything without fatigue—it frees you from tiredness.

Radiancy

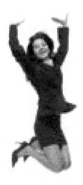

- You're so excited, you can't sit still.

- You receive an unexpected compliment, and you feel a shimmer of delight.

- You're throwing a surprise party for your mom, and she's just about to enter the room.

The excitement, the pleasure, the delightful anticipation, this is the feel of **Radiancy NRG**. It may be small and internal, like the shimmer of delight at a compliment...

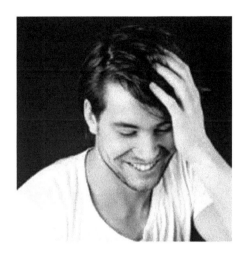

...or it can manifest itself outwardly, like jumping up and down in excitement...

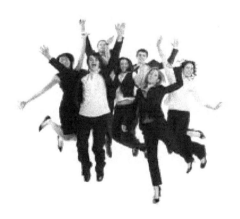

It comes from the body pain reliever of shaking.

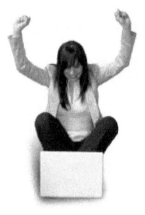

The body feels impulse-charged and actions are spontaneous.

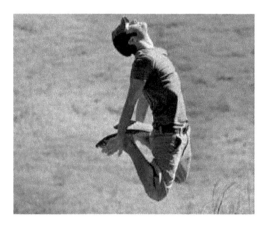

Think back to those audience members who were feeble and stiff when they began to watch the concert, but who were up and dancing by intermission.

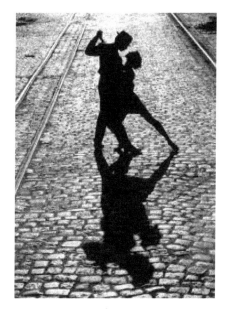

Radiancy NRG did that for them.

The music stirred them inside, they responded with tapping feet, nodding heads, shaking shoulders, and finally with dancing.

...pain disappeared...

Opening a Present

- Imagine you are a child.

- In front of you is a wrapped present. You want to open it, but you have to wait.

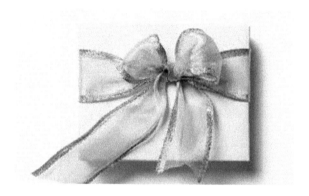

- Finally, it's time! Open it!

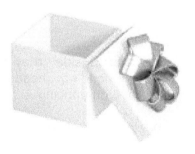

- It's something you really wanted! Let yourself express this in movement...

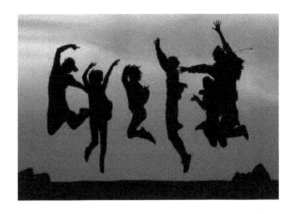

- and in voice...

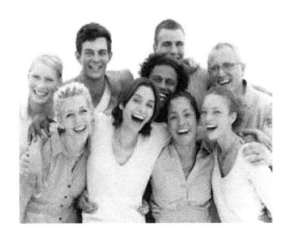

Note inner sensations of anticipation, happiness, excitement, and corresponding outer behaviors, like the gleeful shaking of the body...

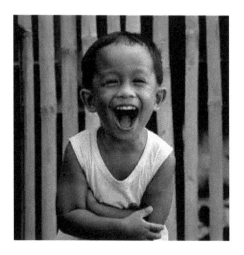

...the whoops of joy, the laughter...

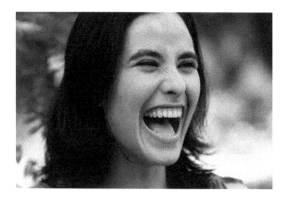

...and the lighting up of the face.

Potency

- You're on a swing, and every pull through your hands and stretch through your legs swings you higher and higher.

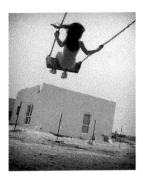

- You lie on your back, lifting a toddler up and holding him in the air while he squeals with delight.

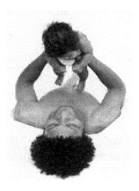

- A succulent piece of fruit seems just out of reach, but by stretching, you get it!

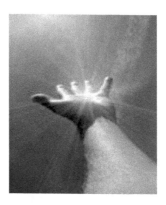

Potency is the organic instruction that evolves from the familiar event of muscle yawning. It allows any physical action to be performed without strain or force. It is a high-voltage muscle yawn that vitalizes the body with a sense of robustness and strength. It relaxes as it empowers, creating optimal efficiency.

The Push Away

- Standing in front of a wall, or a closed door, or even a fence, place your hands on the surface and lean in and then push yourself away from it. Do this several times to feel the sensation of it.

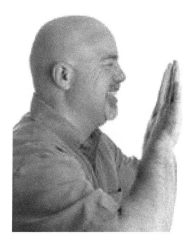

- Now muscle yawn and feel it throughout your back, between your shoulder blades, and along your spine.

- As you yawn, you will feel that your body wants to move away from the surface on which you are leaning, but you won't feel the same effort as you did when pushing with your arms.

- In fact, you will feel as if your back is leading the movement, and you will also feel less of your weight on your hands. Your abdominal area is concaved, while your back is rounded.

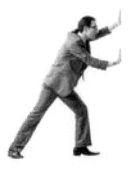

Notice how much easier that feels? You can do lots of these; whereas, when you just push with your arms, your arms can quickly become heavy and tired.

Potency NRG gives us strength and power, but without the force and push often associated with those terms. When you are forcing or straining, your muscles are out of balance, and that is when injury occurs.

Potency protects us from strain and pain. When you use the muscle yawn, the muscles engage as they are meant to do, in the optimal balance between extension and contraction relative to the movement.

Putting it Together

All the different NRG qualities defined here are rarely used to the exclusion of others. They are constantly mingling together in your daily life.

You may be peacefully reading the morning paper, in a state of floating buoyancy, when you see an article that grabs your attention, putting you in a vibratory radiancy state. It might even make you want to take action which could put you into a potency NRG state.

This could all happen in the space of a few seconds. It is more likely, however, that these NRGs don't follow each other sequentially but overlap and occur together.

Thus, when exploring these NRGs, isolate them initially to experience their unique qualities, but recognize their interwoven natures and enjoy the awareness of their presence singly or together.

Walking and Experiencing the Body NRGs

- Find a place where you can walk. As you walk, mix into your walk the now familiar event of each NRG quality: buoyancy, radiancy, and potency *(this can be felt particularly well if you have a slight hill to climb)*.

- Now add to these NRGs the feeling of rhythm in your walk. You can do this by listening to or imagining your favorite music. Allow yourself to move easily in this rhythm. Let your whole body respond.

Can you begin to feel the dance in your walk? Not prescribed dance steps, but your unique personal dance, the physical expression of you in the moment.

What were some of the sensations you experienced?

Lightness?

Looser joints?

Quicker pace?

Confidence?

These are only a few of the healthy results of the Body NRGs at work.

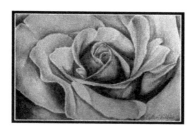

The Vocal NRGs

When you talk, do you feel like you are singing?

Arthur Lessac

Let us agree that any time one engages in playful pitch-change, chanting, or vocal rhythm, he or she is singing. It is our belief that, barring diminished capacity by defect or accident, everyone is capable of singing. Singing is healthy and can:

- Improve your mood
- Relieve stress
- Improve sleep
- Improve posture
- Clear sinuses
- Improve mental alertness
- Boost your immune system
- Increase confidence

Why not realize these healthy benefits when engaged in everyday speech?

It is common for mothers and babies to sing to each other. A baby's developing sense of self and social interaction depends on this exchange, as does the mother's growing understanding of her child's needs.

Toddlers mirror the vocal expressions of others, spoken and sung, which advances social sharing skills and helps in experiencing emotions. Such emotions are recalled later in life when we hear the same chord changes or harmonies in music because singing helps to socialize and can lead to empathy.

Speaking involves pitch, rhythm, and melody—all attributes of singing. We have, at our command, a virtual orchestra, with all the exciting melodies, harmonies, and tonal colors that come with it, giving us the capability for the fullest expression of our inner selves.

The Vocal NRGs offer us the opportunity to experience the many qualities of music that reside within us and the potential for authentic communication with others.

Consonant NRG

When a musician reads a page of music, she doesn't just see symbols; she feels music playing inside of her. To her the symbols represent more than notes—they have:

pitch

duration

rhythm

When orchestrated together they form a musical phrase which expresses a mood or emotion.

Vowels and consonants also have pitch, duration, and rhythm.

When orchestrated together, they form words and phrases that inhabit mood, emotion, and meaning.

Like a musician, we can see beyond the notes and connect with the inherent music of language itself.

We experience most consonants through the sensations of humming and tapping.

Babies can be observed doing both of these actions as they explore the sounds they hear from others and feel the sounds they can make themselves.

Humming

- Close your eyes and hum.

- Feel free to move or sway gently.

- Allow the humming to come close to the sensation of a familiar consonant. A good one to start with is **m**.

- Explore humming on other consonant sounds while moving or swaying your body. Try an **n**. How about a **v**?

- You can hum on:

n m   v z ng l zh th r w y

Notice how each hum has its own quality, some lighter, some darker, some with more buzz, some smoother—all unique.

- Make up your own tunes and melodies with the humming.

When you hum these consonant sounds, you will likely note a pleasant sensation, vibration in the bones of the face and head.

Humming feels good. Allow this vibratory sensation to relax you on the order of internal massage. It revitalizes you.

Tapping

- Begin by tapping as if playing a drum, pretending your finger is a drumstick and the surface on which you are tapping is the drumhead.

- Try doing it very lightly, so that you feel your finger-tap spring away from the surface.

- Explore similar sensations inside your mouth, using your tongue as the drumstick and the hard palate or teeth as the drumhead.

- Settle on a tap you recognize as a consonant. Create a variety of rhythms using that tap.

You can tap on:

p   t   k   g   d   b   ch   dg   ts   dz

The sensation of the spring away action makes them light, crisp, clean, and enjoyable.

You will also note that each tap is unique:

Some have voice (*d* and *g*)

Some do not (*t* and *k*)

Some are like a short hiss (*ch*)

Some pop (*p*)

Combined with their hummed counterparts, they create countless rhythms.

In addition to hummed and tapped sounds, there are voiceless consonant sounds that call forth their own kind of sound effects which also create contrast and variety. They are:

th f h s sh

The beauty of these explorations lies in the discovery of a way of speaking which is no longer merely articulate, but also musical. Musicality enhances intelligibility, interpretation and meaning, along with fluidity and clarity.

It is well-documented that those with disfluency *(those who stutter)* can be fluent when they sing. Those challenged with disfluency tend to triumph with this approach because when consonants are felt as musical instruments, speech becomes music.

Disfluency disappears when the speaker *feels* like he/she is singing, though what is heard is speech.

Musicality makes speaking pleasurable. When speaking is a pleasurable sensation, stress associated with speaking is greatly reduced or eliminated. And that's healthy!

Structural NRG

Structural NRG begins with the familiar event of the muscle yawn. First, let's feel it.

- Open your mouth to say **AH**. Slowly slide from **AH** to **OO** *(as in pool.)*

As you do this, you will note that your side teeth come closer together. By the time you get to **OO**, you may find that the space you felt in the oral cavity when you started has been significantly reduced. The tone may even take on a tinny quality. But does this need to happen?

- Repeat the first action. This time induce a mild, comfortable yawn. Move slowly from **AH** to **OO** without losing the yawn.

Did you notice that you did not have to lose the openness inside your mouth, even on the **OO** vowel, when you added the yawn feel?

The oral cavity becomes a reverse-megaphone shape, with your lips representing the smaller end.

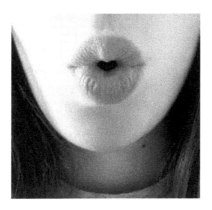

You can feel the cheek muscles naturally reaching further and further forward as you move towards the **OO** vowel. This sensation—the cheek muscles moving forward, the feeling of openness in the oral cavity—is what we call *forward facial orientation.*

The lips and muscles of the face are not pulling backwards towards the ears. Backward movement of the facial muscles while speaking can create tension and strain which interferes with good vocal quality.

Even though you can make the lip opening smaller or larger, the cheek muscles are always gently urging forward. This forward movement, engaged by the sensation of an oncoming yawn and the flexibility of the lips, keep this a comfortable feeling, without a sense of effort to hold it in place.

This is called Structural NRG because the muscle yawn gently urges the cheek muscles forward and creates a structure in which your voice can resonate.

You can feel a lot of yawn or a little bit of yawn, depending upon whether you are talking to someone across the street or standing right next to you.

The point is not to hold onto the yawn in a particular size or shape, but to always feel the energy of it, the feeling of the muscles of the face moving gently, sometimes imperceptibly, forward.

Why is this important? Because the sensation of yawning keeps facial muscles facile and responsive.

You may recall a time when you disapproved of something, or when you were hiding a secret. You may have felt a tightening in your face, particularly around the eyes and mouth, as you tried to conceal your feelings. This kind of tightening can become habitual and eventually interfere with lively, healthy expressiveness.

Structure helps to create optimal space inside your mouth so that you produce a warmer, deeper-sounding tone, without lowering your natural pitch.

You can easily experience this. Cup your hands to your mouth as if you are going to call to someone a distance away.

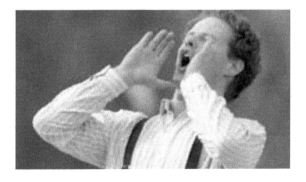

When you call, you will notice that your voice has added depth, even though you are not trying to speak lower or louder. In effect, you have just added with your hands what you could always have naturally with your facial orientation—if those muscles were activated with the slightest sensation of the yawn.

In addition to the positive effects on the quality of the voice, there are other healthful benefits that derive from this forward facial orientation:

- It frees the jaw from tension

- It focuses the voice forward

- It creates ample space for the tongue to operate

- It contributes to the protection and maintenance of dental health by providing a cushion of space between the back teeth, eliminating the tendency to grind

- It provides continuing tension relief for the entire jaw, neck and throat areas, as well as tension relief in the face, chin, head, and shoulders

- It provides good muscle tone in the face, throat, and shoulder areas.

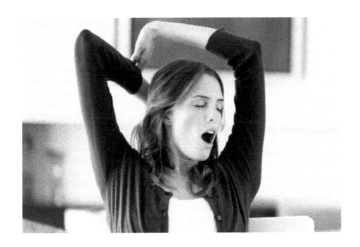

Decreasing the space while still feeling the yawn

Experiment with the following words with the fullest feeling of your forward facial orientation:

ooze
old
all
odd
alms
ounce
add
I'd
oil
snore
earth

- Now try it with these words:

foot
hit
get
just
poor
seer
fair

You probably discovered that the words in the first group were easily recognizable; whereas, the words in the second group were distorted.

Try the second list again. Feel the forward facial orientation, but allow the teeth to come closer together in order to ease any distortion. You don't want to disturb healthy communication.

From Calling to Conversation
Four Levels of Communication

- *(Extravagant)* Explore the first group of words above once more with the full feeling of the facial yawn, as if you are calling out these words from a mountaintop. You'll find you have to speak slowly or else you will pull on your jaw.

- *(Formal)* Explore once again, but this time increase your tempo slightly, while feeling the full facial yawn. It will feel as if you are lecturing to a large group of people.

- *(Informal)* Explore a third time, but now relax the yawn, still feeling slight forward movement of the cheek muscles. Your side teeth will be approximately one finger apart. Imagine you are sitting across a table from a friend, conversing over coffee.

- *(Intimate)* Finally, allow the feeling of this facial yawn to evolve to a subtler state. You increase your tempo to compliment your normal speaking patterns, though a cushion of space should remain fortified by the initial yawn impulse. Imagine that you are sitting next to a friend in a theatre, and you lean in to speak to her so as not to be overheard.

Commitment to the sensation of a full yawn initially will pay off when the space naturally evolves in subtler levels of communication.

Explore all four levels with the following phrases and feel how the interpretation changes:

Oh, no!
Wow!
No more!
It's all over.

Intensify your awareness of this sensation and discover where it occurs spontaneously in your everyday life.

When you talk lovingly to a baby or a puppy, you'll feel yourself using natural forward facial orientation.

When you sip a cup of hot coffee or tea, you'll feel the cheek muscles reaching forward.

Search for other such examples and begin to recognize them as familiar events. When you do, you can easily turn them into organic instructions in order to teach yourself this healthy, flexible facial orientation.

Tonal NRG

When someone speaks lovingly to you, or yells at you, you have a visceral response. Tone of voice provides information and also has a direct physical impact on our bodies.

Hearing a constant angry tone creates anxiety, anger, depression, and withdrawal, all of which poison the healthy body.

Good vocal tone illuminates and warms the inner environment; it is what permits the spirit of respectful communication, even when there is disagreement; and it is like a magnet, drawing people together rather than pushing them apart.

We posit that "tone" is organized vibration and "noise" disorganized vibration. This is why we offer that tone, fundamentally, when felt through the vibration of hard surfaces in the body, has healing properties. Our own self-made tones contain harmonics, or overtones, which, when felt with awareness, lead us to both a sense of calm and centeredness, and to a truer sense of our inner environment, and with that, a recognition of our needs. It allows us to listen to ourselves more deeply than we normally do. Tonal NRG is thus a vibrational therapy.

Wouldn't you like to have a voice that creates good feeling in others and that also feels good to you? This is the healthful choice.

You don't have to go out and get special training to experience this. In fact, you've already experienced the familiar events that will give you the organic instruction for feeling and producing good quality tone.

The Sensation of Tone

- Hum on the **n**. You'll quickly feel a sensation where your tongue touches your gum ridge, and even in the bones of the nose and forehead. These hard surfaces are ideal for transmitting vibrations.

- Say the word **yes**. Pay particular attention to the **y** consonant sound.

- Sustain the **y** consonant in **yes**. It will feel like this: **y-y-y-y-y-y-y-y-y-y-yes!**

- By sustaining it, you hum it, like you did with the **n**. Play with humming the **y** until you can feel the vibrations on your gum ridge, like you felt for the **n**.

Do you notice that when you sustain the **y**, it also sounds like the vowel **EE**?

This is the feel of your voice.

- Without pausing between them, alternate humming the **n** and the **y**.

n-n-n-y-y-y-y-n-n-n-n-y-y-y-y

When you loosen the tongue from the **n**, you feel more sensation/vibration on the gum ridge, right behind your upper front teeth.

- Now add the familiar event of your minimal forward facial orientation, just as if you were gently telling a child **shhhhhh**.

- Body posture helps here. Your head floats up, like a helium-filled balloon, and the rest of your body follows along. Don't lift your chin up or thrust it forward.

Sensation/vibration in the bones of the face and head is the basis of Tonal NRG.

It is a reliable way to create strong, healthy tone without strain or force. What are the health benefits? Natural protection against:

throatiness

vocal fatigue

nasality

denasality

breathiness

The vibrations are both invigorating and relaxing, massage-like, and can therapeutically ease:

pain

anger

strain

distress

pressure

From Humming to Words

The **y** consonant, when sustained, becomes the **EE** vowel and thus is known as a vowel-like consonant. It becomes the bridge between **Consonant** and **Tonal NRG**.

- Hum on the **y** again, feeling the **EE** vowel.

- Once you have found a comfortable, buzzy vibration, experiment with feeling that sensation in these words:

  cheese

  piece

  weepy

  feeling

  creamy

  bleed

- And now into these phrases:

  Please leave me.

  We need this breeze.

  He's a creep.

  Please eat the cheese.

You are experiencing the warm, rich, and easy tone you can use in daily conversation, one that won't be breathy or creaky or disappear at the end of every sentence. In addition, when we want more power without resorting to shouting, this sensation/vibration can evolve into what we refer to as the **Call**.

Calling out to others is a natural and common occurrence in life. Let's explore some calls that might be familiar.

Real Life Calls

In each of these experiments, refresh your feeling of forward facial orientation via the yawn sensation.
.
- You are at a ball game. You are selling popcorn in the stands. Call out *Popcorn* several times.

- You are on a golf course and have just teed-off. Call out *Fore!*

- You are a conductor on a train. It's time to depart. Call out *All aboard!*

- You are a lumberjack and have just felled a tree. Call out *Timber*! Be sure to feel the yawn.

- You are a street vendor, selling strawberries. Call out *Strawberries* so as to attract buyers. Do not frighten them away by shouting—shouting is not calling.

These calls can offer you exhilarating feelings of power without force. Your voice will rise out of you without effort. You may be surprised by the beauty, strength, and effortlessness of your tone.

These situations require the voice to carry over long distances, perhaps even above crowd-noises. Street vendors from every culture use the Call to protect their voices.

Adding more yawn

- You're standing next to a horse you love, and she is very skittish. Calm her by saying, **Whoa, Nellie.**

- Do this again, but this time, experience the forward facial yawn when you say **Whoa**.

- Now, Nellie is harnessed to a small cart and is pulling you along at an easy trot. You need to stop her. Remembering that she is farther away, and that she is not facing you, easily call out **Whoa, Nellie!**

- Repeat this, but again, feel the forward facial yawn sensation when you say **Whoa!**

- Now, Nellie is the lead horse on the stage coach you are driving. There are six other horses. Suddenly, they get spooked and start to gallop. It's a runaway stage coach! You need to get Nellie's attention by calling out **Whoa, Nellie!**

- Repeat the last scenario, and again, when you call, feel the forward facial yawn sensation.

Did you feel the difference between having the yawn and not having it?

If you are feeling the forward facial yawn as we learned it in the Structural NRG section, you will discover that the tones are easy, rich, dark, and full. More importantly, it is effortless.

This is the kind of tone we need for highly emotional situations, such as when we are at the homecoming football game. Its resiliency protects the voice from hoarseness and fatigue.

Emotional Control

Tonal NRG has another important, healthful aspect, though, and that is its effect on your emotions. To the extent that you are able to maintain tonal control in your speech, you will be able to maintain your own equilibrium and reduce disturbing behavior.

If you think back to a time when you have lost control of yourself, you will likely recall that your voice was the first thing to go. When one is angry or upset, it is easy for the voice to become shrill or forced. This results in hoarseness, sore throat, and pain. But if you feel the voice vibrating in the bones of the face or head, you will feel emotion, but it is not likely that you will spin out of control.

Tonal NRG, which cannot function with any kind of force, keeps your voice healthy, and in so doing, keeps you balanced and aware.

Experience the voice with all its musicality:

Consonant NRGs
rhythms and melodies, and

Structural NRGs
open vowels & forward yawn, and

Tonal NRGs
vibratory sensations

make speaking pleasurable. The health benefits of singing are yours every time you speak when you include the vocal **NRGs**.

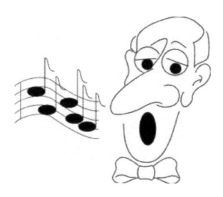

When you talk, do you feel like you are singing?

Part Two: **POWERFUL FEELING**

LOVE, SPIRIT, SOUL

Love is the most melodious of all the harmonies, and we have an innate feeling for it.

Honore de Balzac

Should you go no further in this book, you would benefit from the NRG work you have done. But the body and voice have nothing to express without the natural outgrowth of all that energy into the power of love, spirit and soul.

We have incorporated questions directly from students and workshop participants to help explore the powerful feelings naturally generated by the NRGs. In some cases, we have taken the liberty of combining questions into single queries in the interest of time, space, and the hope that reader-questions would have the best chance of being addressed.

The Body and the Vocal NRGs serve the power poets have throughout the ages assigned to that generated from the beating of the heart. Too often confused with romantic passion and the power of love and energy it produces, *might we continue to use our extension-descriptor* **NRG** *and suggest the presence of* **Love NRG** is sovereign to a far larger domain than to mere romance.

Deborah's story

The best and most beautiful things in the world cannot be seen or even touched. They must be felt with the heart.

Helen Keller

I sat at the bedside of my mother, who was in the late stages of Alzheimer's and had also lost the power to use language. I picked up a magazine and noticed my mother's eyes glance toward it.

Knowing how my mother had loved reading, I put a magazine in front of her and opened it to a page.

There was no response...

I turned pages in my magazine, then in my mother's.

...still no response.

When I next happened to glance up, my mother was staring at me with such intensity I knew something important was happening.

Slowly, without ever losing eye contact, my mother reached out, caressed my shoulder, and said:

You are nice, nice, nice, nice, nice.

Unable to form more words, she held my gaze until the moment had passed and then retreated into her world again. My mother's last hello, our last shared expression of **Love NRG** that had not dimmed despite the loss of her physical faculties.

How grateful I was to have glanced up when I did, for that moment held our last mutual recognition of our love for each other.

It took spirit for her to make that last loving contact. And for a brief moment, I felt our souls had touched.

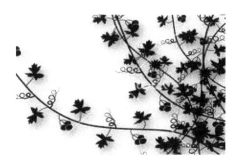

Question:

Is it possible to identify the sensations of Love NRG in the same way that we've been guided to the sensations of Body and Vocal NRGs?

Yes and no. Love NRG is felt in many everyday actions. But the experience is more complex than the Body and Vocal NRGs, and it is experienced differently by each person. Here are some examples of instances where Love NRG is present. Once you discover the sensations of Love NRG, they will trigger greater awareness:

- When you see or interact with a baby.

- When you play with a puppy or a kitten.

- When you take time out of a busy schedule to do something caring for yourself.

- When you burst into song or dance.

- When you do something special for someone else, cook a special meal, make a gift, or help a stranger in need.

- When you cannot wait to begin work in your chosen profession each day.

The Body and Vocal NRGs are *components* of the Love NRG, so when you are feeling them, you are also sensing love.

Question:

I see where those NRGs are engaging in activity that is doing something caring for yourself, but it is there a greater connection?

When you engage in any of the Body or Vocal NRGs, you do something good for your body— you care for it in a loving manner. The connection among NRGs is that they are engaged without force or strain. Should either of those phenomena emerge, you are no longer in the domain of NRG, but are, instead, caught up in the application of effort.

NRG invigorates you; whereas, effort consumes and diminishes energy.

Question:

Do the NRGs proceed in order of greatness or value, first this one, then that one, etc.?

The most beautiful melodies are composed of sound and time, each element thorough in its own virtue, but somehow of greater magnitude having obtained to the greater entity called melody.

Love NRG is the greater entity, or perhaps we can say, the greater station to which the other NRGs obtain.

Love NRG cannot thrive on antagonism, aggression, greed, or on making choices at the expense of others. It is the finest kind of connection with any and all other things because it promotes well-being.

Observation:

Up until we started exploring Love NRG, the other NRGs felt like solid physical sensations. It seems like we've stepped off into another kind of environment, one that is not so concrete, more like metaphysics.

Fair enough. Let's look at that. When learning a skill, it could be writing, drawing, playing a musical instrument, construction, sport, or parenting, each component of the skill possesses virtue that is not quantifiable in the accretion, or accumulation of itself, into the greater entity, the learned accomplishment or undertaking. What, then, is the concrete sensation of which to become aware? It is the sensation of thorough well-being obtained from freedom of effort in the undertaking.

Love NRG flows from the presence of the other NRGs. When in that place where all NRGs are present and engaged, the pervasive sensation of well-being so thoroughly fills experience that it becomes a concrete physical sensation, perhaps not unlike *flow* or *being in the zone*.

Observation:

I can't get past the idea that Love NRG sounds like just another feel-good idea without much basis in fact.

Facts can be concluded from consensus-data in the form of repeated proof protocols relative to theories and pure logic. Facts can also derive from empirical evidence. Put a dozen people in a heated room and only the reality of physical experience will dictate who is or is not comfortable in the room, regardless of the number displayed in the non-subjective, comfort-controlling-data-device, the thermostat.

Key to the notion of empirical experience as evidence is the provable circumstance in which Love NRG can be willfully engaged.

- Imagine you are talking to someone who troubles you in some way. Can you find one or two things about that person that do not trouble you, that provide an opportunity for appreciation?

- Take time to feel the impulse of this sensation and allow it to grow and blossom until it fills you and begins to displace the prior annoyance.

- Imagine yourself again in discussion with this person. Do you find that the things that disturbed you begin to shift or move into perspective and become less irritating?

Appreciation leads to more than mere tolerance for another. With the application of Love NRG, you have created a way to accept which trumps the distortion of critical or negative judgment.
The bounty of Love NRG does not arbitrarily befall you, it does not inure only to a select few,

nor is it of advantage only to those who are lucky. It is repeatable, thus valid in terms of proof, as is the evidence of consensus-data. Perhaps even more so.

Love NRG is the transforming agent of the inner environment, deriving from the consistent engagement of individual NRGs until they become the power of Love NRG which is manifested in the physical sensation of ever more well-being. It is not finite.

Let's look at another real-life situation that we know from looking at the world around us is all too frequent an occurrence.

Imagine you are disturbed by the color of someone's skin.

- Take some time to simply appreciate color as does a painter or an artist. At this point, do not connect it with skin, but simply observe and appreciate the wide variety of shades and hues of color around you.

- Imagine seeing that person again. Note as many colors as you can discover—hair, eyes, vocal tone, and, yes, skin.

- Allow the impulse to appreciate color apart from consideration of another's skin to grow and blossom until you are, again, filled with appreciation such that the distortion of negative judgment begins to be displaced.

- Allow the displacement to proceed until you are transformed by a physical sensation of well-being that acts with the power of a wave of NRG that clears the inner landscape of all vestiges of negativity.

Let's be clear, this is not a superficial and artificially sweetened antidote to the poison of prejudice in its totality.

We are suggesting that in reducing the experience to its most elemental component and in using Love NRG, it is possible to recast the basic response to color as positive, and by extension, perhaps even to a pleasurable acknowledgement of appreciation.

And what is more, it will not take a lot of heavy lifting to project where the recasting of one's responses to such elemental components might lead.

If, after recasting your response to simple color, you still experience a feeling of disturbance with this other person, then you must acknowledge that it has nothing to do with color, and that the reason lies elsewhere.

Calling upon the Love NRG once more, you would then proceed to shift or recast your response to that elemental component of prejudice, until, component-by-component, the feeling of prejudice has been displaced, or diffused.

All other NRGs open the door to awareness of Love NRG. Its warmth enhances even the most minimal intention to create a better life, a better environment, a better world.

When Love NRG grows on the invocation of Tonal NRG, for instance, it leads to a quality of communication that fosters feelings of trust which promote the most positive kinds of engagement from person to person, to community, to society, to country, to culture, to civilization.

Thinking globally or even universally, where might the potential in such a chain reaction end?

Observation:

Just when I begin to grasp the concept of Love NRG, you expand it into something that sounds too grandiose to be believed.

True disbelief, or is it reticence? As with any teaching, readiness and receptivity are all. That you may have resistance to the power of what arises out of the familiar is understandable. What you suspect is too grandiose to be believed has surprised others, as well, in very compelling ways.

Arthur's Story

I conducted an experiment in the early 1940's, a time when African-Americans were forced to use separate facilities, eat at separate restaurants, enter only by back doors, and in general, were treated as less than a lower class, they were a non-existent class in America. A group of young African-American men had been studying with me and had learned to use Tonal NRG.

As an experiment, I arranged for them to meet with a group of young white men, who had no knowledge of the training. The young African-American men were instructed to feel the Tonal NRG, no matter what language they might hear from the white men. All were instructed to talk openly, even to speak as they would on the street. The discussion, which lasted for an hour and a half, was focused on racism and the lack of equality between the two sides.

Arguments occurred, but the African-Americans controlled their anger and recrimination with their Tonal NRG. Although the discussion was at times heated, it never exploded into violence, either physically or verbally.

In the beginning, the white men were combative and rude, but as the conversation evolved, it appeared to me that because the African-American men were able to express themselves without resorting to anger, swearing, or threats, the white men also lost their anger, and listened.

The most telling part of the evening, however, was at the end of the meeting. Both sides stood up and shook hands, and that could have ended it. But one of the white men said, "We still don't agree on many things; but when can we meet again to talk?"

You are in Control

There is no question that the young men in Arthur's story would never have said that they were feeling Love NRG. But their desire to meet again indicated that genuine communication had taken place. The built-in emotional control valve of Tonal NRG opened this doorway, and Love NRG took a step in.

The experiment indicates that communication was at a high level, whereby the young men exhibited heightened perception and awareness in speaking, listening, and in responding. This is Love NRG at work.

   Question:

   Okay, but could the same outcome have occurred without the conscious engagement of Tonal NRG?

There is a chance, of course, but it is far more likely that the two sides would have ended up shouting or perhaps even coming to blows.

The ultimate promise of Love NRG is that each of us has the capacity within us to create high-level communion with others.

It is not necessary to wait for a government or a politician or a spiritual leader to initiate this, for the Love NRG is within each of us, waiting to be utilized.

We are born with it, along with the other NRG qualities; thus it cannot ever leave us. Like all energy, it has no beginning and no ending; it cannot be lost.

Question:

If I am not in the habit of using Tonal NRG, will it still be available to me when it occurs to me to engage it, even after long periods of its not having been used?

If you do not use your voice for a while, Tonal NRG may become rusty—but it would not be gone. Once engaged, it would strengthen and begin to feel good again.

So it is with Love NRG: it does not go away, though it may become rusty. Simply engage and use it, and you will recognize that it is as important to your health and well-being as is the beating of your heart.

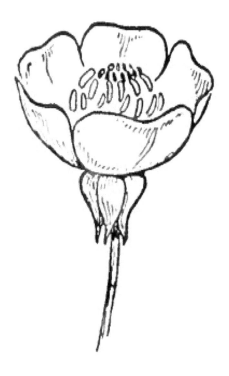

Spirit NRG

Spirit has fifty times the strength and staying power of brawn and muscle.

Mark Twain

You've heard it in phrases like *full of spirit* or *high-spirited* or *that's the spirit!*

You felt it when something *spurred you on* or when you were *on the alert*.

Spirit can be found in something as simple as the joyful laughter of children at play or in something as complex as the taking of a stand against injustice.

Spirit can have many connotations, and the word is often used interchangeably with soul. However, let's make a distinction between the two. For our purposes, **Spirit NRG** has to do with courage, vigor, and vitality. It is not passive.

It is the inner-environmental-electricity that results in a heightened sense of alertness which provides strength of purpose to creative and meaningful endeavor.

Spirit NRG is closely related to Radiancy NRG.

When the announcer at a race cries: *On your mark! Get ready!* potential energy gathers.

When the announcer calls *Go!* it becomes kinetic energy. It gives you power and speed, and perhaps an extra edge.

The musician feels it when the conductor holds up the baton. Again, there is the sense of expectation and potential energy which becomes kinetic when the conductor gives the downbeat.

The radiancy in Spirit NRG acts like a trigger—it gets you going.

Inspiration

Spirit NRG can be felt in inspiration and can lead to creativity, discovery, and adventure. You feel inspiration all the time, though you might not be aware of it.

For example, you are arranging flowers, and you suddenly see that by moving two stems you can create beauty and harmony in the arrangement. You have felt a small burst of inspiration.

Or perhaps you have been working on balancing your checkbook, but the reconciliation eludes you. While reviewing the numbers one more time, you suddenly spot a transposition, or the possibility of success using a different operation.

In no time, reconciliation is achieved. You felt inspiration in that sudden moment of clarity.

Question:

What if there is no one to fire a starting pistol, or to signal the downbeat? How do I find inspiration?

Moments filled with the sensation of inspiration are more plentiful than you might think. They can happen when you view a sunset, a mountain range, or the ocean. Sometimes they occur when you listen to music. It could be the last time you had a great idea and excitedly jumped up and down saying, *Wait! Wait! Listen!*

Observation:

I'm still trying to see how inspiration would be present without there also being success to accompany it.

Let's go back to the familiar. Recall a moment when you did feel inspired. It doesn't matter what the situation was, or what triggered it. *Focus on the physical sensation* that accompanied your feeling of being inspired.

Question:

Is it like a muscle yawn?

Yes, expansion. Do you feel a sense of waking, easing, renewed alertness?

Follow up:

I'm not sure.

Look closer at the physical sensation. Is there a sense of expansion? That is something you can control. It is something you can re-create and allow to grow.

Follow-up:

The physical sensation I have is a desire to laugh.

It's perfectly natural. Allow that desire to grow into robust laughter. Such impulses are material to Spirit NRG. Consider the following quote from one of our workshop participants:

"The body and vocal energies helped me to feel a connection to everyone, because we were encouraged to listen to what was going on not only in ourselves but to everyone around us. There was a fineness of attention which I am not used to in ordinary life activities. Because of this connection and sense of everyone trying something new, I felt part of a supportive group. There was a great deal of laughter from the teachers and this gave us the opportunity to be light in our attempts. Who would ever have thought a sit-up could be so appealing!"

There is a lot of laughter, genuine enjoyment of the work and of each other, in the workshops.

Laughter of this kind is an expression of well-being, and should be welcomed.

Follow-up:

I think I'm laughing because I'm nervous.

Then you are definitely feeling the body pain reliever of shaking! Being nervous happens because we fear something. Fear paralyzes us. The body shakes to free us from this paralysis. Nervous laughter is one result. If you seize this moment to learn from your body's signal, it instructs you to examine the reason behind the nervousness and to deal with the fear. Continued attention to this releases you from the pattern of fear of the unknown, and allows you to *wander in wilderness,* meaning you can approach the unknown with curiosity, rather than with fear.

Any of the body or vocal NRGs can inspire Spirit NRG. We saw this in the case of the young African-American men who were able to navigate contentious waters by investing in Tonal NRG that allowed for communication in a situation which could have escalated beyond confrontation into something other than the positive experience it was. The use of Tonal NRG inspired a growing desire for dialogue in *both* groups.

Follow-up:

Still, it sounds too easy to be as effective as you paint it.

On the heels of significant personal change or transformation, don't we often have the feeling of *But it was so easy!* Or: *Why did it take so long to see it?* Or: *Where has that been?* Authentic insight does not arrive solely on the difficult. The danger is in allowing what comes easily to be taken for granted, or even to be dismissed. When you invest in awareness, the trajectory of all NRGs inspired by such *Ah-ha* moments is outward into the real world.

Investment

- Recall a first-time experience involving something you cared for a great deal; competing in a sport you love; asking someone on a first date; singing solo in front of your church congregation; performing on the stage; perhaps speaking in public on a subject about which you feel passionate.

- As you recall the experience, what do you feel? Excitement? Fear? Butterflies in your stomach? Your heart racing?

What is it that kept you going when your body was saying *run?* You cared! This caring *(Love NRG)* gives you staying power. No matter what challenges you are faced with, your desire to complete the task is greater than your desire to quit. You feel *inspired* with a sense of joy and anticipation in completing the task.

In other words, Love NRG is a strong ally against fear.

Qualities consistent with Love and Spirit NRGs are confidence, readiness, openness, and a willingness to take the risk to sustain an activity. These qualities become the material of courage. When extending one's self beyond what is known, habitual, or comfortable, it likely involves courage.

Courage trumps fear and doubt, which breed inaction. When faced with loss or injury, it is courage that moves you forward, because it is stronger than fear.

When Love and Spirit NRGs are functioning freely, it is an easy step to move from focusing on ourselves to focusing on others.

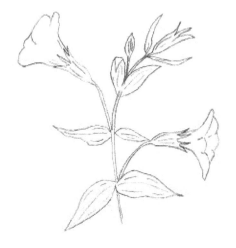

Interinvolvement

As I walked out the door toward the gate that would lead to my freedom, I knew if I didn't leave my bitterness and hatred behind, I'd still be in prison.

Nelson Mandela

Is it possible for one person to change the world? Absolutely! You are changing your world all the time. Before we discuss this, let's quickly review what you've learned:

Energy is the capacity to cause change or to do work. The NRG qualities are identifiable because they cause change in your body.

You feel this change as emotion, heat, movement, vibration, or any number of other words that we use to label these sensations.

Awareness of the sensation of the NRGs allows you to feel both a fundamental NRG, such as *buoyancy,* and the resonance of it, such as *happiness*. Like the ripples that flow from a pebble dropped into water, the results of the NRGs continue to flow into the outer world.

They are the **harmonics** of the NRGs.

Neither the NRGs nor their harmonics contain negatives, they cannot harm you. They are agents for change. When they meet negative forces, they alter those forces and disrupt them.

Awareness of the NRGs and their harmonics is the Feeling Process. It guides you to use the NRGs to remain healthy and to fight the forces that would restrict, defeat, or sicken you.

When you choose to counter a feeling of impatience or irritability with Love NRG, you open the way to feeling kindness and patience. Refusing the restriction of hate with Spirit NRG opens the way to feeling tolerance, acceptance, and interest.

Harmonics such as kindness, patience, tolerance, acceptance, and interest are not passive states. Their vibrations move within us, vibrating at harmonious wavelengths, causing more vibration and still more harmonics. It is a symphony composed and played by you.

This extension of inner energetic motion into the outer environment has a direct effect on those with whom you interact. Thus, the harmonics become evident in your interactions with others.

Action is the result. We call it **Interinvolvement NRG**.

We define this as the mutual exchange of energy between living entities. When you play with a baby, have a heart-to-heart with your spouse, teach a class, or give a presentation to your co-workers, you are engaging Interinvolvement NRG.

Like the body's NRGs, it is free from negatives. Its purpose is to connect you in a positive manner with other living beings. It always results in action, no matter how large or small.

This does not mean that when you engage this energy that everything is smooth sailing. In order to maintain a healthy state of being, you do not allow the reactions of others to contaminate your inner environment. The importance of Interinvolvement NRG is that, regardless of what hurdles may appear on the path, you will respond with power, not with force.

Let's examine this by looking back at the Nelson Mandela quote at the beginning of this chapter. He said: "*I knew if I didn't leave my bitterness and hatred behind, I'd still be in prison*". Mandela made a healthy choice by ridding himself of bitterness and hatred, both negatives to the inner environment because they anesthetize it.

Do you think because he made this decision that every encounter thereafter was full of love and laughter? Of course not. Not only did others not respond in kind, but Mandela must have struggled to stay true to that promise he made with himself.

Nelson Mandela exemplifies the act of choosing repeatedly to respond with Love and Spirit NRGs in all his dealings with other human beings, including those who responded to him with the poison of hatred.

He is revered as a great leader, in large part because he refused to respond from a place of bitterness or hatred, but from love and understanding. His leadership allowed South Africa to rise up out of the ashes of apartheid and in so doing:

He changed the world

Love not hate

Ripples

Harmonics of action

Follow-up:

But I'm no Nelson Mandela! I can't change the world.

Every action you take, however tiny, changes the world.

Mandela once said: "*Having a grievance or a resentment is like drinking poison and thinking it will kill your enemy.*"

Every action we take on the outside is a reflection of our inner environment. If this inner environment is filled with toxins, such as hatred, envy, greed, or the desire to subjugate others, then our actions will contain that toxin, and will contaminate everything and every person with whom we are in contact. Moreover, it will surely contaminate us as well.

By pursuing the body's NRGs and their natural harmonics, you create the climate in which your interactions with others can be free of such toxins, and the actions that ripple out from you will reflect those harmonics and will, by natural extension, have a positive effect in the world.

Follow-up:

Okay, but I don't really think I can be a leader.

Consider this quote from Marianne Williamson *(often mistakenly attributed to Nelson Mandela):*

> *"Our deepest fear is not that we are inadequate. Our deepest fear is that we are powerful beyond measure. It is our light, not our darkness that most frightens us. We ask ourselves, Who am I to be brilliant, gorgeous, talented, and fabulous? Actually, who are you not to be? We are all meant to shine, as children do. It is not just in some of us; it is in everyone and as we let our own light shine, we unconsciously give others permission to do the same. As we are liberated from our own fear, our presence automatically liberates others."*

Or consider these responses from people who have participated in our workshops:

> *"I found and find this focus on the energies and "feelings"...created a human sense of unity regardless of language, heritage or skin color. The inner harmonic sensing helped me tap into my human centre."*

> *"I know that it might sound a bit corny, but I felt like we were just all the same. At the beginning of the workshop there was the usual old judgment of myself and others. By the end of the 10 days it had evaporated. Trust is always a long way off when you have spent a lot of your life being vigilant. Maybe being with others*

who know this too is what makes the Lessac work so liberating."

There are the famous peacemakers, agents of change in the world, like Gandhi, Mother Teresa, Martin Luther King, Jr., and the Dalai Lama.

There are also those who are not so well-known, but who have had an impact on creating a healthier, more humane world: Rosa Parks (Mother of the Civil Rights Movement); John Wallach, (Founder of Seeds for Peace); Peter Benenson, (Founder of Amnesty International).

Some make their mark through writing such as Elie Wiesel, some through entertainment, like Jim Henson.

These people embody the Interinvolvement NRG. They are engaged in a positive manner with other living beings, and their engagement results in positive action.

There are people within your own community, not world-famous, whom you recognize as having a kind of energy that gets things done, makes others feel good about themselves, or calms everyone when tempers rise. Interinvolvement NRG is creating a positive effect in their world, too, whether they are aware of it or not.

One of the strongest calls for Interinvolvement NRG came from Mahatma Gandhi when he said:

"You must be the change you wish to see in the world."

Could you be one of these people? Why not? It is not a matter of money, or opportunity, or anything that the outer environment tells you that you must be or have in order to effect change. Everyone has the capacity to feel the **NRGs**. Everyone has the capacity to effect change.

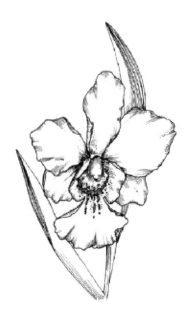

Soul NRG

The living soul of man, once conscious of its power, cannot be quelled.

Horace Mann

Many philosophers have written extensively about the energy of the soul, and we won't presume to come close to their thoughtful ruminations. The question we ask is: Is there a **Soul NRG?** Can we feel it?

Soul has many definitions, including life force, the spiritual part of a person, the emotional part of one's nature, deeply felt emotion, or the embodiment of an intangible quality. These definitions seem to indicate that the soul is felt rather than understood.

Question:

Wait—are you saying now that my soul is tangible?

Not in the sense that you can touch it with your fingers, no. But think back to a time when you had a gut-feeling about something; or maybe you listened to a voice inside.

Was there an accompanying sensation in your heart, your gut, or possibly a prickling at the back of the neck? Let us move forward with the notion that, these sensations are physical manifestations of the movement of the soul— Soul NRG.

Your inner environment is your soul's universe in which Soul NRG becomes the amalgam of all other NRGs, yet more. It is a Gestalt—a unified whole. It strengthens the other NRGs.

For example, Soul NRG raises Love NRG to a higher level of feeling, of experiencing, or of sharing *(soul-mates)*. Soul NRG elevates spirited discussion to communing.

Soul NRG is the source of wisdom. It leads you to the highest level of harmony within yourself and with others. In fact, the Feeling Process is an on-going experience of Soul NRG.

Every time you feel any of the NRGs, you are also feeling Soul NRG.

The information you learn from these NRGs is as valuable to your growth and well-being as the information you learn from books and study. The NRGs keep you healthy on both the physical and spiritual levels of existence.

This is the inner fitness we discussed at the beginning of this book. Remember this?

Yawning relaxes muscles and joints.

Movement is easier.

Posture improves.

Breathing is deeper and more natural.

Organ function improves.

Energy and vitality increase.

Based on what we've learned, let's continue that list:

Increased vitality allows you to enjoy life.

Enjoyment engenders love.

Love invites compassion.

Compassion can lead to empathy.

Empathy can open dialogue.

Dialogue can build a bridge to peace.

A healthy inner life leads naturally to an awareness of your own and others' humanity. This awareness gently guides you toward making a difference in your world.

This work is so simple, and so private, no one else need know you are doing it. By listening to and learning from your body's messages, you grow in awareness of what contributes to your well-being, and what does not. You become acutely aware of toxins and have a way of dealing with them.

The only way to know if this work can have this kind of effect for you is to try it.

As Mandela said, *"One of the things I learned when I was negotiating was that until I changed myself, I could not change others."*

Give yourself this gift of inner health and well-being. Find for yourself the vast source of wisdom contained in your body. Find it through precise sensation and powerful feeling.

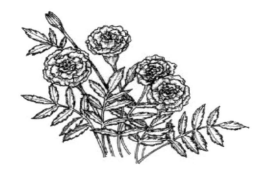

Afterword

What Lies Ahead

I recently returned from teaching two Lessac training workshops in South Africa. Arthur had visited there in the 90's and had always wanted to go back. In fact, he and I had planned to travel to South Africa after we had launched the voice training portion of the Acting, Media, and Culture program at the University of Rijeka in Croatia, where I now sit as I write this. Unfortunately, Arthur did not live to revisit South Africa, passing away shortly after our successful initiation of the curriculum in Croatia. Therefore, it was with a sense of honoring my beloved mentor that I undertook these workshops in South Africa.

But it was also with a sense of adventure. I was getting the opportunity to test whether Lessac training, now called *Lessac Kinesensic Training,* could be applied cross-culturally. I had had some inklings of this when I taught the intensive workshops in America, when we had the occasional foreign student, but this was the first time I would be working with a majority of people for whom English was a second language. I wanted, in my limited time with the participants, to leave them with the knowledge that this training belonged to everyone, not just those who spoke English as a first language and not just to Americans. I taught them in a way that I hoped was accessible, simple, non-competitive, and doable. In other words, I taught them this book.

Throughout his life, Arthur constantly *evolved* his work. He took great pains to choose that word: evolve. He saw "change" as too abrupt. He felt the work would and should always grow, but slowly, since every new idea should be tested over time in the teaching, measuring it against the original principles. That kind of growth, he felt, would eventually evolve Kinesensics in new and exciting ways. I was fortunate enough to be able to watch him teach, discuss concepts intensely with him, challenge his findings, and be a part of the evolution of his work in the last decade of his life.

What is the future of Kinesensics?

Arthur Lessac's work is beginning to grow beyond theater circles, where it began. In the workshops I have led, I have taught teachers and academics, athletes, dancers, ministers, lawyers, business people and politicians, in addition to actors and singers. My students have ranged in age from 5 years old to senior citizens. They come in all shapes and sizes and all degrees of movement and vocal ability. They speak a variety of languages. All are unique in their backgrounds, but they all want the same thing: to express what they feel inside, honestly and without fear. They state this desire in a variety of ways: better articulation, louder or softer voice, higher or lower voice, get rid of nervousness, be able to move away from the lectern, be able to gesture freely, etc. These all point to a desire to communicate; moreover, a desire to be understood.

I have also taught those who work with the voice and body: ESL and TESOL teachers, speech language pathologists, speech therapists, somatic educators, college professors and high school teachers. They, too, have a need to express themselves clearly and to be understood easily. They are also looking for new and effective ways to help their clients/students learn to overcome their obstacles to clear communication.

In order to broaden the scope of the work, the work has to be made available to many more people. Hence this book, which is fashioned so that anyone can experience the essence of the training.

Getting it to more people is one way to grow the work. But it must be grown from within as well. Arthur originally designed the voice work for Americans, at a time when most voice teachers were promoting speech built on British rhythms, phonemes, and intonation. His voice book advocated for a fresh approach to speech training, one not reliant on imitation of another country's language or even of a valued teacher.

Kinesensics honors the individual voice, leading to a democratic way of teaching voice—no one is ever a copy of another, and all are welcomed. This factor has influenced my goals of bringing Kinesensics to other languages. Since all human beings feel all of the energies, the basic principles of the work apply to any language. My recent work in South Africa, and also in Croatia and Puerto Rico, proved this assumption true in Setswana, Afrikaans, Croatian, and Spanish. It has also proved true in Korean, Chinese, and Dutch.

But even more than language skills and expressiveness are the subtle benefits of Kinesensics, which are difficult to quantify, but which affect people deeply. These include confidence, trust, empowerment, calmness, willingness to listen, openness, and joy. Often, these are revealed through testimonials. Here are some:

An Afrikaans woman: *"It was an emotional journey to let go of some of my habitual body and vocal patterns. I grew up thinking that I was expected to be 'cute' and to speak in my higher range. The workshop enabled me to reconsider some of my perceptions about myself and my culture, which made me realize that the body and vocal energies broaden my verbal communicating capacity without taking away from my own identity or culture."*

A Xhosa man: *"In my opinion, the course has been designed to help artists/people in general who do this course to regain the power of the self, and a greater understanding of the power of the body as an instrument. And now I feel closer to who I am."*

Another Afrikaans woman: *"The holistic nature of Lessac teaching means that it can be used as performance training, but is equally relevant to people on a personal level, to help them find their own voice and self-expression. I love the emphasis Lessac training puts on one's inner life. Of everything we covered in these workshops this is the thing that I have been using on a day-to-day level, to help me counteract harmful, self-deprecating or stressful thoughts. I am so grateful that I had this opportunity. It was such an inspiring, empowering and liberating experience. I finished this workshop feeling so much closer to others and myself, and so much calmer in the world. I wish everyone could have this opportunity."*

An Irish man: *"Our group was a mix of nationality, experience and ability, [containing] actors, youth workers and teachers. The striking aspect was to see how everyone moved forward; how everyone's speech was clearer and more full of meaning by the end of our short time together. It's not just for actors; it's for anyone who needs to communicate."*

A Xhosa woman who teaches junior and high school students in one of the most depressed townships in South Africa told us on the last day that she felt empowered, like she had connected with her authentic self. Later, her supervisor wrote, *"[She] has had a complete turnaround and is now the chairperson of a local organizing committee! Total reversal from...before Lessac training - she HAS FOUND A VOICE!"*

These reactions and many others, both verbal and written, confirm for me that this training belongs to everyone. The fact is, with this training, people communicate better, work together better, and are more creative. They are also true projections of their authentic selves, because of what they discover in themselves.

What does this mean? It means that people change their perceptions of each other—they see each other as humans first, cultures second. How they are alike first, how they are different second. This perceptual change has immediate implications that go far beyond what language we speak. How can you hate someone, hurt someone, kill someone, when you see them first as someone like yourself? I am not proposing here that we will wipe out war, hatred, bigotry or killing in a single swoop. But the perceptual shift must be noted; it must be recognized as a beginning, a movement towards openness and trust and away from fear. Fear: the most effective weapon used by those who wish to control others. On a very deep level, Kinesensic training stops fear. This is what I am teaching;

this is how I see the Lessac work continuing to make a significant contribution to the world.

We can all experience this.

It is not about hoping, or wishing, or dreaming. It is right there, inside of all of us, waiting to be discovered, waiting to be explored, waiting to give back to us what we thought we had lost— our true selves.

Deborah Kinghorn
June 15, 2013
Rijeka, Croatia

Lightning Source UK Ltd.
Milton Keynes UK
UKHW02f2014030518

322082UK00010B/730/P

9 780988 498211